Hormone Reset Diet Meal Plan

Complete 30 Day Meal Plan On How To Reset Your Hormones

Introduction

Reset your hormones naturally with the teachings in this book to experience weight loss and other benefits you've never thought possible!

Have you ever tried to lose weight but you simply couldn't lose any?

Well, here is a shocker.

Sometimes being overweight has nothing to do with calories and exercise!

It's no wonder why more than half of Americans are on some kind of diet or exercising plan-even as the rate of obesity keeps rising each year.

The problem with a huge number of us is we have misfiring hormones, which make it impossible for us to lose weight no matter how hard we try. What this means is that your hormones may be sabotaging or working against all your weight loss efforts, which means you will just be going round in circles if you don't do something different. As such, if you've been trying to lose weight unsuccessfully, perhaps what you need is a new approach to weight loss.

You can't continue doing the same things you've been doing over the years (without any fruit) and expect different results, right?

Obviously, there is no factory reset button in your body where you get to reset your hormones and other body systems!

What then?

As you well know, we are what we eat. This means if you can do something about your food, you can fix your hormones as well.

This sounds interesting and promising, right?

This dietary approach to fixing your hormones is called the hormone reset diet. With a hormone reset diet, the goal is to balance your hormones, so that they stop pulling you behind in your weight loss efforts and instead provide a favorable environment for you to burn fat and keep it that way!

And if you are wondering how to go about resetting your hormones, this book has everything you need to do just that.

By reading this book, you will get to learn what the hormone reset diet is, how it came to being, how it works and how you can adopt it. The book will then walk you through a 30 day meal plan with a wide range of delicious recipes that you can use to reset your own imbalanced hormones.

To be more specific, you will learn:

- What it means for your hormones to be out of balance

- **What signs you may exhibit if your hormones are out of balance**

- Which hormones actually go out of balance and why they matter so much

- **How to reset each of the key hormones that control many of the busy processes**

- How to use food to make that happen

- **Foods you should be eating and those you should be avoiding while on an hormone reset diet**

- A 30 day meal plan set out in an easy to grasp format

- **And much, more!**

Let's begin!

Table of Contents

Introduction _____ **2**

An Introduction To The Hormone Reset Diet For Complete Beginners _____ **8**

   Brief History Of The Hormone Reset Diet? ____ 9

   How Do Hormones Affect Your Weight Loss? __ 10

The Place of Hormones In The Weight Loss/Gain Equation _____ **12**

How Does The Hormone Reset Diet Work? 16

   So, How Do You Adopt The Hormone Reset Diet? _____ 23

Hormone Reset Diet Recipes _____ **33**

Breakfast Recipes _____ **33**

   Vanilla Green Milkshake _____ 33

   Vegan Chickpea Omelette _____ 35

   Pumpkin Porridge _____ 38

   Baked Avocado And Egg _____ 40

   Chocolate Cherry Smoothie _____ 42

   Teff Bowl With Chia Jam _____ 44

Vegan Sandwich With Tempeh Bacon _____ 46

Banana Reset Shake _____ 49

Reset Crab Cakes _____ 50

Green Smoothie _____ 52

Hormone Reset Brownies _____ 54

Lunch Recipes _____ **56**

Beet And Carrot Salad _____ 56

Quinoa Salad _____ 58

Chilled Herb And Cucumber Soup _____ 61

Raw Sweet Potato And Carrot Salad _____ 63

White Bean And Veggies _____ 65

Southern Caesar Salad _____ 66

Cashew Broccoli Noodles _____ 69

White Beans With Roasted Fennel _____ 71

Vegan Sauerkraut Soup _____ 73

Oven Roasted Vegetables With Herbs _____ 75

Dinner Recipes _____ **77**

Thai Salmon _____ 77

Skillet Mushroom Chicken And Quinoa _____ 79

Veggie Pizza With Sunflower Seed Cheese ____ 82

Portobello Mushrooms Steak _____ 84

Artichoke And Spinach Risotto _____ 86

Shakshuka _____ 88

Avocado With Quinoa And Sautéed Greens __ 90

Moroccan Miso, Lentil And Pumpkin Soup __ 92

Instant Pot Bison And Cabbage Stew_____ 94

Buddha Bowl _____ 96

Conclusion _____ **98**

An Introduction To The Hormone Reset Diet For Complete Beginners

If this is your first encounter with the hormone reset diet, you must be wondering what hormone reset diet is.

So what is it?

Let me explain that:

The hormone reset diet was discovered and created by the Harvard educated physician called Dr. Sara Gottfried. As the name suggests, the hormone reset diet is a diet or a way of eating that aims at resetting your seven metabolic hormones that need to be balanced for you to lose weight and live a healthy life.

Basically, what this diet does is that it cures your hormone imbalance by helping your body grow new receptors for your seven metabolic hormones namely cortisol, estrogen, insulin, leptin, growth hormone, testosterone and thyroid. That automatically balances your hormones and puts your body in a position to lose weight fast and efficiently.

But where did the hormone reset diet come from?

Here is a brief history of how this diet was discovered and created.

Brief History Of The Hormone Reset Diet?

Well, the story of the hormone reset diet starts with its founder Dr. Sara Gottfried. Dr. Sara Gottfried is a physician whose expertise is in the category of a woman's body and everything that can go wrong with it. In her field of work, she dealt with a lot of weight loss issues. In fact, she used to counsel women all day long on how to lose weight.

Here is a shocker though; at 39 Dr. Sara was struggling with her own weight. She went from one diet to another but she couldn't lose her weight. So she decided to visit her doctor and seek advice. The response that she got is what everyone gets told when they visit the doctor, 'eat less and exercise more' and that's when it hit her that maybe her weight loss issue or lack of thereof had nothing to do with calories or exercise. Having been in the medical field, she knew she had been truly been following the rules that she would otherwise be telling her patients so she knew her weight had to have another cause.

Dr. Sara got this strong hunch that the problem could be hormonal. So she went on and tested her hormones and found out that her cortisol (the stress hormone) was three times what it should have been. After that discovery, she went on a three weeks journey of trying to reset her hormones and guess what; she surprisingly started losing weight and she knew she was on to something.

What happened next is Dr. Sara decided to take on the top seven hormones (estrogen, insulin, leptin, cortisol, thyroid, growth hormone and testosterone) that fluctuate or are imbalanced when you can't lose weight and created a program where people could work on balancing those hormones. That is how the hormone reset diet was discovered.

The question that might be going on in your mind is:

How Do Hormones Affect Your Weight Loss?

From time in memorial, we have been told that what counts when it comes to weight loss is your calories and your activity levels. What you were never told is that hormones count more.

Why?

This might come as a surprise to you but hormones regulate your cravings, appetite, metabolism and body shape in a way that calories and exercising can't. In fact, the first sign that you get when you have a hormone imbalance is gaining weight. This is because 99% of weight gained is usually hormonal –but a lot of people don't connect the dots. You don't understand that most of your problems with your mood, feelings of being fatigued, depression and energy fluctuations are all related to your hormones.

In short, hormones have the ability to keep you from the body that you want.

But how do hormones manage to do that-block you from losing weight? Let me explain that next.

The Place of Hormones In The Weight Loss/Gain Equation

Well, there are so many factors that contribute to hormones going bad but here are the three major contributing factors to your hormones going bad that automatically encourages difficulty in loss of weight.

1. ## *Excessive stress*

One of the worst things you can go through when trying to lose weight is being excessively stressed. This is because excessive stress brings imbalance to your hormones.

But how does it do that?

An increase in stress usually leads to an increase in a hormone called **cortisol.** What you may not know is that cortisol is a stress hormone that promotes the conversion of blood sugar into fat.

So when its level increases in your body, you automatically become a fat storing machine, as your body only focuses on storing your blood sugar as fat.

The thing is; when you are in that situation where your body is focused on storing fats, it is impossible for you to lose weight no matter how much you diet or exercise.

This is because for any amount of weight your workouts will help shed off, your body will bring it back through the process of fat storage. In short, it will be like trying to fill a tank with water when the tank has several holes; no matter how much you try, you will never be able to fill it. That is one reason why you are not losing weight.

2. *Exposure to toxins*

The majority of the population in the world today is exposed to toxins each and every day. Some of the common toxins we are exposed to include genetically modified foods, herbicides that we use on our farms, pesticides that we spray in our houses, the air pollution from cars, prescribed drugs, beauty products like lipstick and the list goes on and on.

What you need to be aware of is that when we are exposed to the just mentioned toxins, we usually absorb them and once they are in our body, they act like the **hormone estrogen**.

What that does is that it increases the level of estrogen in your body. That increase then causes what we call **an estrogen overload,** which means you have too much estrogen in your body.

An overload in estrogen is said to promote or encourage insulin insensitivity, which means your body becomes prolific in storing energy for fats than using them for energy. This automatically adds you weight because your body turns into a fat storing machine that only focuses on adding you weight. Just like with excessive stress, that process makes it hard for you to lose weight.

3. *Consuming too much sugar*

The other way that your hormones can block you from losing weight is when you consume too much sugar.

Let me explain.

One type of sugar that our bodies get when we consume food is fructose. Fructose is normally found in processed foods and most fruits.

The truth is; fructose is good for your health when you consume the recommended five daily servings per day.

But as you are well aware, nowadays, the five daily servings contains more fructose than what the body can utilize, which means a lot of us consume excessive fructose and that's where the problem comes in.

The consumption of excessive fructose usually forces your liver to convert them as fat and sending them in your bloodstream as triglycerides since your liver can't deal with the fructose fast enough to utilize as energy. The rise in triglycerides leads to an increase in the level of your **hormone leptin**.

Leptin is the hormone that tells to stop eating because you are full. Unfortunately, when there is too much leptin in your system, your body becomes resistant to leptin and its message. This means your body becomes unable to get the 'stop eating you are full' message. This automatically leads to weight gain no matter how much you try losing weight.

In conclusion, when your hormones are imbalanced, you usually store extra fat regardless of whether you are exercising, dieting or not. This is why bringing the balance back into your hormones is the most powerful bio-hack for your weight, energy and your health in general.

So how can you fix your imbalanced hormones and get to enjoy better supply of energy, efficient weight loss, controlled mood and better health in general? By simply following the hormone reset diet. But how does it work? The answer lies in the next chapter below.

How Does The Hormone Reset Diet Work?

One thing that Dr. Sara learnt in her experiment with hormones is that hormones are responsible for a lot of body functions so when they 'malfunction', a lot of our bodily functions go wrong too.

That said, Dr. Sara could have easily turned to prescribed hormone replacement medicine or therapy but she didn't. Instead, she worked hard to find a natural way of correcting hormonal imbalance and that's how she came up with the 21-day hormone reset diet-which corrects hormone imbalances through changing your eating lifestyle.

So how does the 21 day hormone reset diet work?

The hormone reset diet is an eight step process that seeks to balance seven hormones.

The first seven steps of this diet involve you eliminating a certain food group in each of the seven hormones to resynchronize your wrecked metabolism. Let's now break down the seven steps that you need to follow to reset your hormones.

Step 1: Reset Estrogen

The first step in the hormone reset diet is to balance your level of estrogen.

How does that work?

The hormone reset diet makes you eliminate the one group of food that brings estrogen imbalance in your body and that is meat-red meat to be precise.

You might not know this but the cows that we get our meat from are nowadays given the hormone estrogen by their owners for the purpose of encouraging growth in the cow.

So when you eat meat, that estrogen is transferred to your body where it increases the level of estrogen. This leads to you having an overload of estrogen- and as you saw in the previous chapter, this normally leads to you having trouble losing weight.

So the first step of hormone reset diet helps you reset estrogen by making you go meatless for three days- which is the period your body needs to correct the imbalance in estrogen.

That said, that's not the only food that you are supposed to eliminate in step one.

The other food product is alcohol.

Step 2: Reset Insulin

The second step in the hormone reset diet concentrates on balancing your insulin.

What does insulin have to do with weight?

Insulin is an important hormone in your body because it helps you convert food into energy. That said, insulin can easily turn from being helpful to being harmful to your body when its levels in your body are excessive.

Basically, what happens when you have a high level of insulin in your body is you develop insulin resistance where insulin is unable to transport glucose to your cells. When that happens, glucose builds up in your blood stream, which leads to diabetes and other health issues like inflammation. Excessive levels of insulin also hinder you from losing weight because they turn your body into a fat storing machine, as you saw in the previous chapter.

This step balances your insulin through restricting you from consuming sugar and sugary products-the culprits that raise your insulin levels.

Step 3: Reset Leptin

As you saw in the previous chapter, the hormone leptin is usually imbalanced by excessive consumption of fructose. So the third step that you are going to take is to eliminate the high fructose fruits from your meals. The diet allows you to replace them with fruits like avocados and olives, as they fare much better with your hormones. The other alternative is you can limit your fruit intake to 2-3 servings per day.

Step 4: Reset cortisol

As you now know cortisol is a stress hormone that encourages your body to store fat. When you have high levels of cortisol in your body, it becomes very hard for you to lose weight.

So what promotes cortisol in your body? The answer is coffee and caffeine in general.

So in this step, you are prohibited from using coffee for three days, which helps your cortisol to reset and come back to its normal levels.

Step 5: Reset Thyroid

The fifth step in the hormone reset diet is to eliminate grains from your food.

Grains like potatoes, pastas, white rice and breakfast cereals might seem yummy to consume but what you don't know is the gluten that you get from grains can be mistaken for your thyroid tissue once they get to your body.

What that does is that it leads to an autoimmune response, which can cause serious problems like inflammation, irritable bowel syndrome and possible cancer.

Worst of all is the imbalance in your thyroid makes it hard for you to lose weight.

Step 6: Reset growth hormone

In step 6, you cut off your consumption of dairy.

Why is this important?

This is important because the world we live in today has exposed us to dairy products that came from livestock, which have been injected with several growth hormones for the purpose of making to produce more milk. Therefore, by consuming milk that has traces of the growth hormone, we end up introducing these hormones in our body systems.

In this step, you eliminate dairy products from your meals and maybe replace them with non-dairy milk and other products like coconut milk or almond milk.

Step 7: Reset testosterone

As you saw in the previous chapter, we as human beings are affected by toxins and artificial chemicals each day. This exposure to toxins sometimes makes you insensitive to insulin and leptin.

The toxins also expose you to other forms of chemicals called the androgen disruptors which lower testosterone in men and raise it in women.

The effect of that is usually a testosterone imbalance in your body, which leads to frequent colds, achy joints and fatigue. The imbalance also hinders your weight loss efforts.

Common sources of toxins include cosmetics, hygiene products and foods which have chemicals.

Step 8: Fixing your metabolism for good

Those seven steps that you have just learnt above help your body balance your misfiring hormones within a period of 21 days or after dealing with each hormone for three days.

Therefore, at this stage, your body is in sync with your hormones. In other words, your hormone imbalance is now healed and that's where step 8 comes in.

Step eight is meant to help you fix your metabolism issue once and for all.

How does it do that?

It does that by helping you find your personal food code.

Let me explain.

The seven steps that you have undergone asked you to eliminate at least 8 groups of foods. The truth is; some of the foods you have eliminated are healthy to your body and a good number of them don't cause hormone imbalance in your body.

So for that reason, step eight makes you go through a process of re-introducing the suspect foods that you had eliminated but in a one by one method.

The idea here is, when you are in sync with your hormones, you can detect food sensitivities when you reintroduce your eliminated foods- and all you have to do is for example eat meat and try to observe how you feel. If your energy level goes down and you are unable to lose weight, you will know that you are sensitive to meat and eliminate it forever from your meals. After that, you will go to the next food you had eliminated.

So start trying the foods that you eliminated from the meat to dairy products. Observe how you feel when you eat each food type. If you are energetic, your health is good and you are able to lose weight, the type of food you ate should be introduced to your diet. But if the food you reintroduce leaves you sick and energy deprived, then you should know that's the food that causes hormone imbalances in your body and you can go ahead and keep it completely off from you meals.

At the end of this process, you will have come up with your customized diet or way of eating that does not cause an hormonal imbalance.

So, How Do You Adopt The Hormone Reset Diet?

To adopt this diet, you will need to follow three simple steps.

Here they are:

1. Know What To Eat And What Not To Eat

As you now know, the hormone reset diet balances your hormones through food. So the first step that you need to take when adopting this diet is to know what you should eat and what you shouldn't eat.

What to eat

The foods that you should eat are basically whole organic foods.

This includes most vegetables and fruits like avocado, flaxseed, chia seeds and whole grain like quinoa, brown rice, buckwheat, unsaturated oil and fats like canola oil, most nuts, olive oil and lean protein from wild caught fish, eggs and chicken breasts. Those are some of the foods that you are allowed to eat. That said, the list of the foods to eat is usually long and the other way you can know what to eat is by you learning what you shouldn't eat and eat everything else that is not on that list.

What not to eat

In the first 21 days, you will need to stop consuming dairy foods, gluten, sugar, alcohol, most oils, caffeine, processed foods, saturated fats, full-fats, fried foods, artificial sweeteners and red meat.

After the 21 days, the foods that we have highlighted above stop being off the limits completely. After that, you can minimize their consumption or get rid of them depending on how your body will react during the food re-entry process.

2. Go Out For Shopping

Now that you know what to eat and what not to eat, you need to visit your kitchen and get rid of the foods that are not hormone reset diet friendly. You should then make a shopping list and go out to shop for new stock.

Here is a good example of a shopping list you can make:

Beverages

- Water
- Unsweetened almond or coconut milk
- Herbal tea

Pantry items

- Nuts and seeds like raw almonds, cashews, chia and flax seeds
- Coconut, olive and avocado oil

Fridge and freeze items

- Organic and free range eggs

- Organic chicken
- Organic and free range turkey
- Organic and free range chicken
- Cold water fish

Fresh produce

Here, you can buy your favorite vegetables that are organic, locally grown and preferably in season.

Good examples of such foods include:

- Carrots
- Celery
- Cabbage
- Beets
- Asparagus
- Broccoli
- Kale
- Spinach
- Arugula

Your favorite herbs

- Tarragon
- Parsley
- Cilantro

Your favorite low fructose foods, which are organic and locally grown:

- Avocados
- Olives
- Coconut
- Berries
- Lemons

3. Make a meal plan

With a meal plan, you will know beforehand what you are going to cook and perhaps prepare it earlier so that you don't fall into the temptation of eating something that will offset your hormones again before you are done resetting them fully in the 21 days.

This list is important because it gives you a sense of what you will need in a week or in a month time, which helps you to shop accordingly.

Here is the 30 day meal plan that I promised you earlier:

Hormone Reset Diet Meal Plan

Days	Breakfast	Lunch	Dinner
1	Vanilla green milkshake	Roasted vegetables with herbs	Thai salmon
2	Vegan chickpea omelette	Vegan sauerkraut soup	Skillet mushrooms chicken and quinoa
3	Pumpkin porridge	White beans with roasted fennel	Veggie pizza with sunflower seed cheese
4	Baked avocado and egg	Cashew broccoli noodles	Portobello mushrooms steak
5	Chocolate cherry smoothie	Southern Caesar salad	Artichoke and spinach risotto
6	Teff bowl with chia jam	White bean and veggies	Shakshuka

Hormone Reset Diet Meal Plan

7	Vegan sandwich with tempeh bacon	Raw sweet potato and carrot salad	Avocado with quinoa and sautéed greens
8	Banana reset shake	Chilled herb and cucumber	Moroccan miso, lentil and pumpkin soup
9	Reset crab cakes	Quinoa salad	Instant pot Bison and cabbage stew
10	Green smoothie	Beet and carrot salad	Buddha bowl
11	Reset brownies	White bean and veggies	Veggie pizza with sunflower seed cheese
12	Pumpkin porridge	Southern Caesar salad	Portobello mushrooms steak
13	Teff bowl with chia jam	Cashew broccoli noodles	Artichoke and spinach risotto

Hormone Reset Diet Meal Plan

14	Chocolate cherry smoothie	White beans with roasted fennel	Shakshuka
15	Baked avocado and egg	Chilled herb and cucumber	Thai salmon
16	Vegan chickpea omelette	Raw sweet potato and carrot salad	Skillet mushrooms chicken and quinoa
17	Vanilla green milkshake	Vegan sauerkraut soup	Veggie pizza with sunflower seed cheese
18	Green smoothie	Quinoa salad	Artichoke and spinach risotto
19	Reset brownies	Beet and carrot salad	Shakshuka
20	Pumpkin porridge	Southern Caesar salad	Avocado with quinoa and sautéed greens

Hormone Reset Diet Meal Plan

21	Vegan sandwich with tempeh bacon	Roasted vegetables with herbs	Moroccan miso, lentil and pumpkin soup
22	Teff bowl with chia jam	White beans with roasted fennel	Instant pot Bison and cabbage stew
23	Reset crab cakes	White bean and veggies	Buddha bowl
24	Banana reset shake	Roasted vegetables with herbs	Veggie pizza with sunflower seed cheese
25	Baked avocado and egg	Vegan sauerkraut soup	Portobello mushrooms steak
26	Reset brownies	Beet and carrot salad	Thai salmon
27	Vegan chickpea omelette	Raw sweet potato and carrot salad	Skillet mushrooms chicken and quinoa

Hormone Reset Diet Meal Plan

28	Green smoothie	Chilled herb and cucumber	Veggie pizza with sunflower seed cheese
29	Vanilla green milkshake	Cashew broccoli noodles	Portobello mushrooms steak
30	**Reset crab cakes**	Quinoa salad	Instant pot Bison and cabbage stew

Now that you have the meal plan, it's now time for you to learn how you can prepare the foods in the above meal plan.

Learn that in the next chapter.

Hormone Reset Diet Recipes

In this chapter, you will discover some of the delicious hormone reset diet recipes that you can use when you adopt the hormone reset diet.

Breakfast Recipes

Vanilla Green Milkshake

Serves 2

Prep time: 5 minutes, Total time: 5 minutes

Calories: 520, Proteins: 12g, Carbohydrates: 72g, Fats: 22g

Ingredients

4-6 pieces of dinosaur kale, with stems removed

1/2 avocado

2 scoops of reset 36 0TM All-In-One Shake

Unsweetened hemp, coconut or almond milk

2 tablespoons of chia seeds (should be soaked for four hours in an unsweetened hemp, coconut or almond milk)

Handful of ice

Directions

Place all the ingredients in a blender. Pulse until everything is well mixed.

Serve in a glass and enjoy.

Vegan Chickpea Omelette

Serves 2

Prep time: 10 minutes, Cook time: 5 minutes, Total time: 15 minutes

Calories: 144, Proteins: 9g, Carbohydrates: 18g, Fats: 4.5g

Ingredients

For stuffing

1 tablespoon of cilantro

¼ cup of small broccoli florets

¼ cup of chopped tomatoes

2 minced garlic cloves

¼ red onion chopped

For the chickpea batter

¼ teaspoon of sea salt to taste

¼ teaspoon of baking soda

¼ teaspoon of onion powder

¼ teaspoon of garlic powder

¼ teaspoon of turmeric powder

2 teaspoon of nutritional yeast

2 teaspoon of apple cider vinegar

3/4 cup plus 1 tablespoon of unsweetened non-dairy milk

¾ cup of chickpea flour

Directions

Make chickpea batter by whisking all the chickpea ingredients in a Pyrex measuring cup. The batter should be like pancake batter- easy to pour and not too thick to stir. Set aside to allow the batter to sit.

Sauté red onion together with garlic in a heated non-stick skillet until browned. Add broccoli to soften. Place the broccoli on a plate.

Return the broccoli back to the heated skillet. Add olive oil. Pour half of the batter into the pan and add in garlic, onions, broccoli and tomatoes. Give the mixture 2 minutes to bubble up and firm along the edges.

Gently fold over one side of the batter and cook for another one minute. Cover the non-stick skillet with a lid and turn off the stove to let the mixture steam for about 5 minutes.

Garnish the mixture with lime wedges, sliced avocado, minced red onion and more tomatoes. Add sea salt and pepper to taste.

Serve and enjoy.

Pumpkin Porridge

Serves 1

Prep time: 2 minutes, Cook time: 13 minutes, Total time: 15 minutes

Calories: 527, Proteins: 17.15g, Carbohydrates: 18.18g, Fats: 44.95g

Ingredients

1 tablespoon of pumpkin seeds

Stevia to taste, optional

1-4 tablespoons of non-dairy milk of choice

1 teaspoon of cinnamon

1/3 cup of pumpkin puree

1 tablespoon of cashew butter or almond butter

1 tablespoon of ground cashews

3 tablespoons of ground hemp seeds

1 tablespoons of ghee or butter

Directions

In a small pot over low heat, heat the ghee.

Add all the other ingredients using as much non-dairy milk as you need to get your preferred consistency.

Cook the porridge gently over low heat. Let the porridge heat up until everything is heated through.

Top the porridge with pumpkin seeds.

Serve on a bowl and enjoy.

Baked Avocado And Egg

Serves 2

Prep time: 5 minutes, Cook time: 18 minutes, Total time: 23 minutes

Calories: 222, Proteins: 8.5g, Carbohydrates: 7.9g, Fats: 18.5g

Ingredients

Fajita seasoning or your favorite seasoning

Pepper and salt to taste

1 egg

1 halved organic avocado with pit removed

Directions

Start by preheating the oven to 425 degrees Fahrenheit.

Flip the avocado side over and then slice off a sufficient amount of the rounded skin for the avocado to sit flat when the fleshy side is up.

In a baking pan, place the avocados fleshy side up. Add salt into each hole.

Prepare the egg mixture. Whisk the egg in a bowl.

Divide the egg mixture between the avocado holes. Season the avocado with salt and pepper.

Place the baking pan on the oven and bake it for 16- 18 minutes or until the egg is fully set.

Serve the baked avocado and egg. Eat with a spoon.

Chocolate Cherry Smoothie

Serves 2

Prep time: 10 minutes, Total time: 10 minutes

Calories: 284.6, Proteins: 12.5g, Carbohydrates: 54.4g, Fats: 6.1g

Ingredients

1/2 teaspoon of cinnamon powder

1 teaspoon of lemon or lime juice

1 teaspoon of vanilla extract

A handful of dry cherries (they should be pre-soaked in hot water for 10 minutes)

A handful of hazelnuts, pre-soaked overnight

A handful of pumpkin seeds

1 tablespoon of coconut butter

2 tablespoons of raw unsweetened cacao

1 avocado

Directions

Add all the ingredients in a blender and blend them together until smooth.

Serve in a glass and enjoy.

Teff Bowl With Chia Jam

Serves 1

Prep time: 5 minutes, Total time: 5 minutes

Calories: 54.2, Proteins: 0.2g, Carbohydrates: 13.5g, Fats: 0.2g

Ingredients

1 tablespoon of nut butter of choice

½ tablespoon of chia seeds

A fistful of fresh raspberries

1/2 teaspoon of ground cinnamon

1 tablespoon of milled flaxseeds

50 grams of teff grain

1/2 cup of dairy-free coconut yogurt

Directions

Pour the coconut yogurt in a bowl and add in teff, flaxseeds and cinnamon.

Give them a good mix.

Transfer the mixture into a jar to stand overnight.

Prepare the chia jam the next day. Mash raspberries with chia seeds and let them sit for 5 minutes.

Spoon the chia jam onto the teff. Add a generous spoon of nut butter. Serve and enjoy.

Vegan Sandwich With Tempeh Bacon

Serves 2

Prep time: 10 minutes, Cook time: 30 minutes, Total time: 40 minutes

Calories: 450, Proteins: 18g, Carbohydrates: 48g, Fats: 15g

Ingredients

1- 2 tablespoons of almond butter

¼ avocado

2 sliced whole grain English muffins.

1/2 teaspoon of olive oil

1 1/2 cups of torn/chopped kale

¼ teaspoon of black pepper

½ teaspoon of garlic powder

1 teaspoon of smoked paprika

1/2 tablespoon of liquid smoke

2 tablespoons of maple syrup

¼ cup of avocado or olive oil

¼ cup of low-sodium tamari or soy sauce

8 ounce of package of tempeh

Directions

Start by cutting tempeh into ¼ inch thick slices/strips.

In a shallow dish, add in paprika, liquid smoke, maple syrup, oil, tamari, pepper and garlic powder.

Use a fork to whisk the mixture together. Add in tempeh slices. Cover the dish, place it in the fridge and let the mixture marinate for 1 hour or up to 3 hours.

Preheat your oven to 400 degrees Fahrenheit.

In a baking sheet that is lined with parchment paper, arrange the tempeh slices in a single layer.

Add in any marinade that was leftover over the tempeh.

Place the baking sheet in the oven and bake for 15 minutes.

Remove the baking sheet from the oven, toss the tempeh and bake it for another 5- 10 minutes or until the tempeh becomes crispy.

As the tempeh bakes, you can be preparing the kales.

In a skillet, over medium heat, add in oil and kale.

Sprinkle some salt and pepper and let the kale cook until the kale gets crispy and the kale is bright in color. This will take you 5 minutes.

Toast your English muffins.

Once done, lay the avocado on one half and sprinkle it with a small amount of sea salt.

On the other half, spread the almond butter.

Lay down the kale and 3 -4 pieces of sliced tempeh bacon- on top of the avocado. Top the sandwich with the almond butter.

Repeat the process to make another sandwich.

Banana Reset Shake

Serves 2

Prep time: 5 minutes, Total time: 5 minutes

Calories: 252, Proteins: 5g, Carbohydrates: 65.2g, Fats: 0.8g

Ingredients

1 tablespoon chia seeds

1 frozen banana, peeled

20 ounces of cashew or almond milk

2 tablespoons of natural peanut butter

2 scoops of warrior blend vanilla

Directions

Combine all the ingredients in a blender and blend them for 30 seconds or until everything is smooth.

Serve in a cup and enjoy.

Reset Crab Cakes

Serves 4

Prep time: 5 minutes, Cook time: 20 minutes, Total time: 25 minutes

Calories: 100, Proteins: 19g, Carbohydrates: 9g, Fats: 17g

Ingredients

3-4 tablespoons of coconut oil or ghee

½ teaspoon of black pepper

½ teaspoon of garlic powder

½ teaspoon of paprika

1 teaspoon of dried parsley

1/2 teaspoon of rosemary salt

1/2 pound of fresh crabmeat, fully cooked

2 eggs

1 clove of fresh garlic

1 small shallot

4 radishes

Directions

Start by placing garlic, shallot and radishes in a food processor. Pulse until everything is finely minced.

In a large mixing bowl, add the eggs and beat them. Add in garlic, shallot and minced radishes. Mix in the crabmeat together with the spices.

In a large frying pan, over medium heat, heat the coconut oil or ghee.

Use your hands to form small flat cakes with the crab mixture. Fry the cakes with each taking approximately 5-7 minutes on each side. Or fry until the sides turn browned and are well cooked through.

Serve and enjoy.

Green Smoothie

Serves 2

Prep time: 2 minutes, Cook time: 2 minute, Total time: 4 minutes

Calories: 174, Proteins: 9.7g, Carbohydrates: 18.3g, Fats: 8.3g

Ingredients

1 fresh or frozen ripe banana

1 teaspoon of coconut oil

2 teaspoons of chia seeds

2 teaspoons of raw Maca powder

2 teaspoon of raw spirulina

1 tablespoon of raw sesame seeds

2 tablespoons of hulled hemp seeds

2 cups of water

Directions

In a blender, add in hulled hemp, sesame seeds and water. Process the ingredients on a high speed for one minute to get raw milk.

Add in banana, coconut oil, chia, maca and spirulina. Process the mixture for a further one minute on medium speed. The mixture should be well incorporated.

Serve on a glass and enjoy.

Hormone Reset Brownies

Serves 4

Prep time: 15 minutes, Cook time: 1 hour, Total time: 1 hr. 15 minutes

Calories: 129, Proteins: 1.62g, Carbohydrates: 21.26g Fats: 4.68g

Ingredients

1 cup of unsweetened pure cacao powder

1 tablespoon of baking powder

1- 2 tablespoons of sorghum flour

½ cup of avocado oil

½ cup of coconut sugar

½ cup of organic, hardwood-derived xylitol

2 large eggs

2 medium sweet potatoes

For icing

¼ cup of organic, hardwood-derived xylitol

2 dark chocolate bars (should be 85% pure cacao or higher)

Hormone Reset Diet Meal Plan

Directions

Start by preheating your oven to 350 degrees Fahrenheit.

In a large pot, add 6 cups of water and bring them to a boil.

Use a peeler to peel sweet potatoes. Cut each potato into several large pieces. Add the potatoes to the boiling water and let them cook for 30 minutes or until they are tender.

Drain the water and mash the potatoes in a large bowl using a fork.

Stir in cacao powder, baking powder, sorghum flour, avocado oil, coconut sugar, xylitol and eggs.

Transfer the batter into a greased 8 by 8 inch baking dish. Bake for 20- 25 minutes.

As the cakes bake, you can be making the icing. Place the chocolate bars in a microwave and melt them. Stir xylitol into the melted chocolate.

Once the brownies are done, remove from the oven and pour the melted chocolate over them to form a thin even layer. Give the brownies a few minutes to cool. Serve and enjoy.

Lunch Recipes

Beet And Carrot Salad

Serves 4-6

Prep time: 10 minutes, Total time: 10 minutes

Calories: 71.9, Proteins: 1.8g, Carbohydrates: 3.8g, Fats: 1.5g

Ingredients

For the salad

1/4 cup of chopped fresh flat-leaf parsley

1/4 cup of chopped scallions

1 cup of chopped raw walnuts

2 cups of shredded carrots

2 cups of peeled and shredded raw beets

For the dressing

1 teaspoon of salt

1 teaspoon of ground cumin

2 tablespoons of apple cider vinegar

¼ cup of freshly squeezed orange juice

Zest of one orange

½ cup of extra-virgin olive oil

Directions

Start by preparing the salad. Use a large bowl to combine all the salad ingredients.

Prepare the dressing. Place all the dressing ingredients in a jar. Cover with a lid and shake the mixture until everything is well combined.

Add the dressing to the salad and toss the mixture until well coated.

You can keep the salad in the fridge for later or serve at room temperature.

Quinoa Salad

Serves 4

Prep time: 10 minutes, Cook time: 55 minutes, Total time: 65 minutes

Calories: 280, Proteins: 12g, Carbohydrates: 39g, Fats: 9g

Ingredients

4 sliced scallions

½ teaspoon of cinnamon

½ teaspoon of ground cumin

¼ teaspoon of ground black pepper

¼ teaspoon of salt

4 teaspoons of apple cider vinegar

1/3 cup of pine nuts

3 tablespoons of extra virgin olive oil, divided

1 medium sweet potato that is peeled and cut into ½ inch cubes

1 cup of rinsed quinoa

Hormone Reset Diet Meal Plan

Directions

Start by preheating your oven to 400 degrees Fahrenheit.

Prepare your quinoa: Combine a mixture of quinoa and 2 cups of water in a small saucepan over medium heat. Bring to a boil and let the quinoa simmer until all the water has evaporated. That will take 15 minutes. Turn the heat off. Cover the saucepan and let and the quinoa sit for at least one hour.

Prepare the sweet potato: Add 1/2 tablespoon of olive oil in a roasting pan. Place the sweet potato cubes on the pan and toss the two ingredients together. Let the potato bake for about 25 minutes or until the potato cubes can be pierced with a fork. Set aside.

Prepare the pine nuts: In a small pan placed over medium heat, add pine nuts and let them toast lightly. Stir them regularly. Set aside.

Prepare the vinaigrette: Place the remaining three tablespoons of cinnamon, cumin, pepper, salt, vinegar and olive oil in a small bowl. Whisk the mixture well. Set aside.

Once the quinoa dries up, use a whisk to break apart its seeds. Place the seeds on a large bowl. Add 1/2 of the vinaigrette and use the whisk to mix everything together. If you like your quinoa very wet, you can add in some more vinaigrette.

Combine the foods. Add in pine nuts, sweet potatoes and scallions into the quinoa bowl and mix gently.

Serve on a plate and enjoy.

Chilled Herb And Cucumber Soup

Serves 2

Prep time: 30 minutes, Total time: 30 minutes

Calories: 86.6, Proteins: 6.3g, Carbohydrates: 6.8g, Fats: 3.8g

Ingredients

Radishes, edible flowers, fresh herbs, zucchini noodles, avocado and sprouts to garnish

Sea salt and pepper to taste

4 cups of chopped English cucumber

1 cup of packed baby spinach

1/2 cup of chopped and packed dandelion greens

1/2 cup of chopped cilantro

1/2 cup of chopped parsley

1/4 cup of lemon juice

2-4 cloves of garlic

2 tablespoons of extra virgin olive oil

Directions

In a blender, combine everything except the garnish ingredients. Blend the ingredients until smooth. Taste the mixture and adjust the seasoning as preferred.

Transfer the mixture in a jar and place it on the fridge to chill for 15 minutes or for up to a few days.

Remove from the fridge and pour into two bowls. Garnish the soup with zucchini noodles, herbs, avocado and sliced radishes and enjoy.

Raw Sweet Potato And Carrot Salad

Serves 2

Prep time: 20 minutes, Total time: 20 minutes

Calories: 136.7, Proteins: 1.9g, Carbohydrates: 22.8g, Fats: 4.6g

Ingredients

1/3 cup of pine nuts

2 tablespoons of organic virgin olive oil

1/ 2 lemon

1 orange

½ grapefruit

2 large carrots

1 large sweet potato

Directions

Start by peeling both the potato and the carrots. If the carrots are organic, just leave them unpeeled.

Make small spaghetti type of swirls of the potato using a spiralizer or a mandolin. Use the same mandolin to slice your carrots thinly and add them in your salad bowl.

Juice the pulp of the orange and grapefruit together with the juice of zest. Pour the juice over the sweet potato and carrot mix.

Add in the Himalayan salt and olive oil and mix. Place the bowl in the refrigerator and let it marinate for one hour as you turn it after every 20 minutes.

Sprinkle the pine nuts over the salad and serve.

Hormone Reset Diet Meal Plan

White Bean And Veggies

Serves 1

Prep time: 10 minutes, Total time: 10 minutes

Calories: 360, Proteins: 10g, Carbohydrates: 30g, Fats: 13g

Ingredients

Freshly ground pepper and salt

1/4 teaspoon of kosher salt

2 teaspoons of extra-virgin olive oil

1 tablespoon of red-wine vinegar

1/2 diced avocado

1/3 cup of canned white beans, rinsed and drained

3/4 cups of veggies such as cherry tomatoes and chopped cucumber or any veggies of your choice

2 cups of mixed salad greens

Directions

In a medium bowl, combine avocado, beans and veggies.

Drizzle the veggies with oil and vinegar and then season them with salt and pepper. Toss the mixture to combine.

Serve the greens on a plate and enjoy.

Southern Caesar Salad

Serves 3

Prep time: 15 minutes, Cook time: 10 minutes, Total time: 25 minutes

Calories: 41, Proteins: 2g, Carbohydrates: 2g, Fats: 3g

Ingredients

For the Caesar dressing

1 tablespoon of lemon juice

1- 2 teaspoons of minced garlic

1/2- 1 teaspoon of anchovy paste

1/4 teaspoon of pepper

1/4 teaspoon of fine kosher salt or sea salt

3-4 tablespoon of avocado or olive oil

1/2 tablespoons of honey mustard

1 egg yolk

For the bowl

1/2 cup of sliced zucchini

1 cup of chopped cherry tomatoes

1/2 cup of toasted gluten-free bread crumbs

1/2 teaspoon of paprika

Lemon wedge

1 cup of green peas, lima beans or black-eyed peas, canned or cooked and drained

5-6 cups of chopped mustard greens

1/2 cup of chopped onions

1 teaspoon of avocado or olive oil or clarified butter

For the toppings

Tabasco

Lemon wedges

Crushed red pepper flakes

Garlic powder to taste

Grated parmesan cheese

Directions

For the Caesar dressing

In a medium bowl, whisk together a combination of lemon juice, garlic, anchovy paste, pepper, salt, oil, honey and mustard and egg yolk until the mixture is creamy.

For the bowl

On a sauté pan over medium to medium high heat, heat the oil. Add in onion and stir fry it until fragrant.

Add in a splash of lemon, peas, mustard greens, paprika and sea salt. Toss the mixture and then cover the pan with a lid. Let the food steam for five minutes. Once done, place the greens in a large bowl.

Add in toasted gluten free bread crumbs, zucchini and cherry tomatoes. Toss the greens with the Caesar dressing.

Top the salad with the optional grated Parmesan and sprouts. Season the salad with garlic, salt and pepper to taste. Sprinkle the salad with the crushed red pepper flakes and drizzle with Tabasco and lemon.

Serve in a plate and enjoy.

Cashew Broccoli Noodles

Serves 6

Prep time: 25 minutes, Cook time: 5 minutes, Total time: 30 minutes

Calories: 270, Proteins: 8g, Carbohydrates: 20g, Fats: 7g

Ingredients

All natural hot sauce

2 tablespoons of fresh lime juice

2 cloves of minced garlic

3/4 cup of unsalted cashews

4 green onions that are thinly sliced diagonally

2 cups of sugar snap peas, trimmed and cut into matchsticks

1 red bell pepper, trimmed and cut into matchsticks

5 cups of broccoli florets, cut into 1 inch pieces

1 ½ tablespoons of peeled and grated fresh ginger

2 tablespoons of coconut sugar

3 tablespoons of divided grape seed oil

3 tablespoons of natural unsalted creamy peanut butter

3 tablespoons of reduced sodium tamari

2 12-ounce of packaged kelp noodles (you can alternatively use brown rice or mung bean noodles)

Directions

Start by soaking kelp noodles in warm water for about 5 minutes to partly soften. Drain the noodles and then cut them into pieces you can manage.

Prepare the sauce. Whisk ¼ cup of water, ginger, and sugar, 1 tablespoon of oil, peanut butter and tamari together in a small bowl. Set aside.

Place a large heavy-bottomed pot on high heat. Heat 2 tablespoons of oil. Add bell pepper, broccoli and cook for 1 minute as you stir regularly. Add peas and cook for a further one minute. Add garlic, cashews and onions and cook for 30 seconds as you stir constantly. Then proceed to mix in the noodles and cook for a further minute. Stir the sauce in and let the mixture cook for the final minute.

Remove the vegetables from the heat and straight into a large bowl. Sprinkle the food with lime juice and toss to combine. Enjoy as a salad or wrap in romaine lettuce and have it with hot sauce and a squeeze of lime juice.

White Beans With Roasted Fennel

Serves 8

Prep time: 14 minutes, Cook time: 20 minutes, Total time: 34 minutes

Calories: 70.8, Proteins: 1.1g, Carbohydrates: 7.3g, Fats: 4.7g

Ingredients

4 cups of fresh baby spinach

2 15.8 ounce can of great northern beans

3 tablespoons of grated Parmigiano-reggiano cheese

Cooking spray

2 minced garlic gloves

¼ teaspoon of ground red pepper

½ teaspoon of salt, divided

¾ teaspoon of freshly ground black pepper

3 tablespoons of olive oil

4 cups of thinly sliced fennel bulb

Directions

Preheat your oven to 450 degrees F.

In a large bowl, combine garlic, red pepper, ¼ teaspoon of salt, ½ teaspoon black pepper, 1 tablespoon of oil and fennel. Toss for the fennel to coat well.

In a baking sheet coated with cooking spray, arrange the fennel mixture in a single layer. Place on the oven and bake until the fennel starts to brown or for 15 minutes. Remove from the oven and stir as you sprinkle cheese evenly over the fennel mixture. Return to the oven and bake until brown or for 5 minutes.

Place a large non-stick skillet over medium heat and heat the remaining 2 tablespoons of oil. Add beans and cook for 2 minutes. Add the funnel mixture, ¼ teaspoon of salt, ¼ teaspoon of black pepper and funnel mixture. Cook for 2 minutes and then serve immediately.

Vegan Sauerkraut Soup

Serves 8

Prep time: 20 minutes, Cook time: 25 minutes, Total time: 45 minutes

Calories: 59.6, Proteins: 2.2g, Carbohydrates: 5.4g, Fats: 4.5g

Ingredients

Sea salt and pepper to taste

1 bay leaf

1 15-ounce can of white beans, drained and rinsed

2 cups of water

8 cups of low sodium vegetable broth

2-3 cups of sauerkraut drained and rinsed

1/4 cup of quinoa, uncooked and rinsed

3 medium potatoes, peeled and chopped into ½ inch cubes

2 medium carrots, thinly sliced

1 medium onion, finely diced

1 rib celery, finely diced

Directions

Place a large pot over medium heat. Sauté onion and the finely chopped celery with a small amount of water or vegetable broth for 5 minutes or until it has softened and is golden.

Add in water, broth, bay leaf, quinoa, potatoes and sliced carrots. Bring the mixture to a boil. Reduce the heat to let the mixture simmer for 15 minutes or until the veggies are tender.

Add sauerkraut to the vegetables. Add white beans with their juice and let the vegetables cook for a further 10 minutes.

Remove the bay leaf and pour half the soup into the blender. Blend until it's smooth. The soup should be slightly cooled when you pour it into the blender. Transfer the soup back to the pot and stir. You can also use immersion blender to cream a part of the soup.

Season the soup with salt and pepper to taste.

Serve and enjoy.

Oven Roasted Vegetables With Herbs

Serves 4

Prep time: 10 minutes, Cook time: 35 minutes, Total time: 45 minutes

Calories: 88, Proteins: 2g, Carbohydrates: 11g, Fats: 4g

Ingredients

1 teaspoon of black pepper

1 teaspoon of Himalayan pink salt

1 teaspoon of dried oregano

2 tablespoon of extra virgin olive oil

1 ½ cups of Vidalia onion

1 cup of Brussels sprouts, sliced

1 ½ cups of medium zucchini, sliced

1 ½ cups of yellow squash, sliced

1 ½ cup of eggplant, sliced

Directions

Start by preheating your oven to 350 degrees F.

Piece all the vegetables to be ¼ inch in thickness and toss them lightly with olive oil.

Line your baking sheet with parchment paper. Arrange the vegetables on the baking sheet. Place it in the oven and roast for 20 minutes.

Remove the baking sheet from the oven. Season the vegetables with oregano, salt and pepper. Make sure the vegetables don't start to brown too quickly. If they do, cover them with a foil.

Return the baking sheet to the oven and roast for another 15 minutes or until tender.

Remove from the oven. Serve on a plate and enjoy.

Dinner Recipes

Thai Salmon

Serves 4-6

Prep time: 15 minutes, Cook time: 15 minutes, Total time: 30 minutes

Calories: 574.9, Proteins: 79g, Carbohydrates: 3.6g, Fats: 25.1g

Ingredients

3 minced garlic cloves

1/2 medium red onion, sliced thinly in half rings

1 tablespoon of freshly grated ginger

2 tablespoons of toasted sesame oil

2 tablespoons of fish sauce

2 tablespoon of lime juice

3 tablespoons of coconut aminos

4 tablespoons of sesame seeds

Grated rind of 1 lime

2 pounds of wild salmon filets

Directions

Preheat your oven to 350 degrees Fahrenheit.

Put the salmon, with the skin down, in an oiled glass baking form. Then zest the lime into a mixing bowl before adding all the other ingredients.

Pour the zest mixture over the salmon. Cover the salmon with aluminum foil but make sure it does not touch the salmon.

Bake the salmon for 15 minutes or until it is just cooked.

Slice the salmon into pieces and serve it over brown rice or buckwheat.

Skillet Mushroom Chicken And Quinoa

Serves 4-6

Prep time: 10 minutes, Cook time: 15 minutes, Total time: 25 minutes

Calories: 341, Proteins: 26g, Carbohydrates: 37g, Fats: 11g

Ingredients

¼ cup of freshly grated parmesan

1 tablespoon of chopped fresh thyme

4 cloves of minced garlic

¼ teaspoon of black pepper

24 ounces of cremini baby bella mushrooms

1/2 teaspoon of divided kosher salt

1 pound of boneless skinless chicken breasts, cut into 1 inch cubes

2 tablespoons of divided extra virgin olive oil

1 cup of uncooked quinoa

2 cups of low-sodium chicken stock

Directions

Use a medium sized skillet placed over low heat to bring 2 cups of chicken stock to a gentle boil.

Add quinoa and let it boil for a few minutes before you reduce the heat to let it simmer.

Cover the skillet and let cook for 12- 15 minutes or until the liquid is absorbed.

Place the skillet aside. Let it cool for 10 minutes or until the remaining liquid is completely absorbed. Fluff the quinoa with a fork and set aside.

Place a skillet over medium high heat. Heat 1 tablespoon of olive oil. Sauté the chicken as you season it with ¼ teaspoon of kosher salt for 4-6 minutes or until the chicken is no longer pink.

Transfer the chicken to a plate lined with paper towels. Wipe the skillet clean with a paper towel. Add the remaining 1 tablespoon of olive oil and heat it over medium high heat. Add black pepper, salt and mushrooms. Cook until the mushrooms start to brown or for 3 minutes as you stir occasionally.

Add in garlic and continue cooking until the mushroom is tender and has lost its liquid or for approximately 4 minutes. If there is still some liquid left in the pan, increase the heat and let it cook until almost all the liquid disappears, which might take you one minute.

Stir in thyme, ¼ cup of parmesan cheese, chicken and quinoa. Serve the mushroom warm with some sprinkle of parmesan.

Veggie Pizza With Sunflower Seed Cheese

Serves 4

Prep time: 10 minutes, Cook time: 10 minutes, Total time: 20 minutes

Calories: 148.1, Proteins: 4.1g, Carbohydrates: 11.6g, Fats: 9.7g

Ingredients

For the pizza

1 large tomato, sliced

1 cup of sliced mushrooms

1 yellow or red pepper

12 mixed olives

Salt

Garlic powder

Oregano

Extra virgin olive oil

1 1/2- 2 tablespoons of tomato paste

Plain store-bought pizza base

For the sunflower seed cheese

1 ½ tablespoon of nutritional yeast

1/2 teaspoon of garlic powder

2 tablespoons of extra virgin olive oil

1/3 teaspoon of salt

2 teaspoons of lemon juice

1/2 cup of water

1/3 cup of sun flower seeds

Directions

Preheat your oven to 400 degrees Fahrenheit.

Spread the tomato paste evenly on your pizza base. Sprinkle some oregano, garlic powder, a bit of salt and olive oil.

Prepare the sunflower seed cheese. Use a blender to blend all the ingredients of the sunflower seed cheese until you form a smooth paste. Spoon the paste onto the pizza base.

Slice up two closed cup mushrooms and add to the pizza. Add 1 large ripe tomato, pepper and olives. Sprinkle the pizza with some oil and a dash of sea salt.

Put the pizza in the oven and let it cook for 10 minutes.

Serve and enjoy.

Portobello Mushrooms Steak

Serves 2

Prep time: 5 minutes, Cook time: 20 minutes, Total time: 25 minutes

Calories: 118, Proteins: 11g, Carbohydrates: 16g, Fats: 11 g

Ingredients

2 large whole Portobello mushrooms

A dash of ground black pepper

1/2 teaspoon of dried basil

1 teaspoon of dried thyme

1/2 tablespoon of tomato paste

1/2 tablespoon soy sauce

1 tablespoon of mirin or sherry

3 tablespoons of balsamic vinegar

1 large garlic clove, minced

1/ 2 small yellow onion diced

1/2 cup of vegan beef broth or vegan vegetables

1 tablespoon of vegan butter

Directions

Heat butter over medium heat in a large frying pan. Once the butter is melted, add in half broth and bring to a simmer. Add in garlic and onion. Let the broth cook for 8 minutes over medium high heat.

As the broth cooks, lay all the remaining ingredients in a small bowl, excluding the remaining broth and mushrooms- and whisk them together. Use a damp cloth to wipe, clean and pull off the mushroom stems.

Add the whisked mix to the pan. Reduce the heat to medium. Bring the mix to a simmer. Add in the Portobello caps and their stems. Cover the pan and cook for about 8 minutes. Turn the mushrooms gently and add the broth that had remained. Let the mushrooms cook for 8 minutes.

Serve while hot and top with juice and onions. Enjoy.

Artichoke And Spinach Risotto

Serves 4

Prep time: 5 minutes, Cook time: 25 minutes, Total time: 30 minutes

Calories: 365, Proteins: 13g, Carbohydrates: 30g, Fats: 16g

Ingredients

1 tablespoons of chopped parsley

2 tablespoons of nutritional yeast

¼ teaspoon of black pepper

½ teaspoon of sea salt

1 tablespoon of lemon juice

1/2 cup of raw cashews soaked in water overnight

2 cups of spinach

1/2 cup of diced artichoke hearts

4-5 cups of vegetable stock

¼ cup of dry white wine

¾ cup of Arborio rice

1 cup of thinly sliced snap peas

2 tablespoons of finely diced green garlic

1 finely chopped onion

1 tablespoon of olive oil

2 tablespoons of vegan butter

Directions

Place a stockpot over medium heat. Add oil and vegan butter and let them heat up. Sauté the onion until translucent and then add in garlic and sauté for a further 30 seconds.

Add rice and snap peas and let cook until the rice starts to toast and brown slightly. Add in wine to deglaze pan.

Add ½ of the stock at a time as you stir frequently until all the stock has been absorbed and the rice is cooked. When the food is halfway cooked, add spinach and artichoke hearts so they can cook into the rice slightly.

In a high speed blender, add 1/2 cup of broth, lemon juice and cashews. Blend the combination until smooth.

Add the cashew cream slowly into the cooked rice. Add nutritional yeast, pepper and sea salt. Let the food simmer to combine.

Top the meal with parsley and serve while hot.

Shakshuka

Serves 4

Prep time: 5 minutes, Cook time: 40 minutes, Total time: 45 minutes

Calories: 795, Proteins: 55g, Carbohydrates: 59.5g, Fats: 37.7g

Ingredients

4 eggs

1 cup of shredded kale or spinach

¼ cup of water

Sea salt and black pepper

1 teaspoon of paprika

1 teaspoon of ground cumin

1 teaspoon of harissa sauce

1 tablespoon of tomato paste

1 crushed garlic clove

1 tin of canned tomatoes

1 chopped tomato

1 medium eggplant, chopped

1 chopped red capsicum

1-2 teaspoon of coconut oil

Directions

Start by preheating your oven to 180 degrees Celsius.

Place a medium frying pan over medium heat. Heat the oil and add in eggplant and capsicums. Cook the capsicum for 5-10 minutes as you toss frequently until they are soft.

Add in water, pepper, sea salt, paprika, cumin, harissa, tomato paste and tomatoes. Let them simmer for 10-15 minutes or until the sauce becomes thick. Stir in the spinach or the shredded kale in the last minute.

Transfer the sauce into a baking dish. Gently make four hollows at the top and crack the eggs straight into the holes. Place the baking dish into the oven and bake until the eggs are cooked to your liking. This usually takes 10-15 minutes.

Serve in a plate and enjoy. Alternatively, serve with a sprinkle of fresh herbs and a dollop of yogurt.

Avocado With Quinoa And Sautéed Greens

Serves 2

Prep time: 5 minutes, Cook time: 5 minutes, Total time: 10 minutes

Calories: 472, Proteins: 11.2g, Carbohydrates: 50.6g, Fats: 27.4g

Ingredients

Sea salt to taste

½ lemon juiced

1/8 teaspoon of cayenne pepper

Handful cilantro

¼ red onion finely diced

1 avocado, peeled halved and pitted

For the greens

Coconut oil or butter for frying

1 handful of soft herbs

1 handful of spinach or chard

1 handful kale

Serve with

1 cup of cooked quinoa

Directions

Heat a small quantity of butter or coconut oil in a pan. Add the greens and sauté over medium heat until soft.

Add lemon, cayenne, cilantro, onion, avocado and salt and pepper to taste in a mixing bowl. Give them a good mix and then toss in cooked quinoa -to heat the greens slightly.

Serve in a plate and top with smashed avocado.

Moroccan Miso, Lentil And Pumpkin Soup

Serves 2

Prep time: 5 minutes, Cook time: 40 minutes, Total time: 45 minutes

Calories: 1154, Proteins: 37g, Carbohydrates: 134g, Fats: 46g

Ingredients

3 tablespoons of olive

3 tablespoons of white miso paste

1/3 cup of lentils or split peas

1 ½ teaspoons of cumin seeds

1-inch piece ginger, thinly sliced

1 cinnamon stick

1 finely chopped chilli

1 finely chopped garlic

1 diced onion

2 coarsely chopped carrots

3 pounds of seeded, peeled and chopped pumpkin

Directions

In a pan placed over low heat, cook onion, garlic and salt. Stir frequently as you cook until soft or for 3 minutes. Add the spices and let cook until fragrant.

Stir in pumpkin, split peas and carrots to coat in the onion mixture.

Add six cups of water into the saucepan. Bring the vegetables to a boil then let them simmer until split peas are soft. That will take you 30 minutes.

Remove the cinnamon stick from the soup. Blend the soup until smooth.

Allow the soup to cool to about 176 degrees Fahrenheit and then slowly stir in miso paste. You shouldn't heat miso over 176 degrees because the beneficial bacteria will be lost.

Serve in a bowl and top with roasted seeds, anise and sprouts.

Instant Pot Bison And Cabbage Stew

Serves 4

Prep time: 10 minutes, Cook time: 40 minutes, Total time: 50 minutes

Calories: 113.3, Proteins: 13g, Carbohydrates: 13.4g, Fats: 1.5g

Ingredients

2 tablespoons of coconut aminos

6 cups of chicken or vegetable stock

2 tablespoons of finely minced ginger

Hot sauce, chilli flakes or ground black pepper to garnish, optional

3 cloves of minced garlic

1 medium yellow onion, chopped into thin slices

3 medium carrots, peeled and sliced into rounds

½ savoy cabbage, shredded

1 tablespoon of extra virgin oil

1 pound of ground bison

Directions

Set the instant pot to sauté. Add in oil together with onion, carrot and cabbage. Let the mix sauté as you stir regularly for 5 minutes.

Add in bison. Let it cook for 3 minutes before you turn off the sauté mode.

Add coconut aminos, chicken stock, ginger and garlic. Lock the instant pot lid and make sure the valve is sealed.

Turn on the soup mode on the instant pot and let the vegetables cook for 30 minutes. Once cooked, use the quick release to let the pressure out.

Taste and adjust salt and aminos as required.

Garnish the food with pepper and serve while hot.

Buddha Bowl

Serves 2

Prep time: 25 minutes, Total time: 25 minutes

Calories: 500, Proteins: 20g, Carbohydrates: 55g, Fats: 25g

Ingredients

½ cup of canned chickpeas, rinsed

½ cup of cooked quinoa

1 ½ cup of baby kale

1 teaspoon of za'atar

1 minced clove of garlic

1 tablespoon of lemon juice

2 tablespoons of tahini

3 tablespoons of hot tap water

¼ teaspoon of divided salt

½ teaspoon of ground cumin

1 teaspoon of extra virgin olive oil

1 cup of small cauliflower florets

Directions

Preheat your oven to 425 degrees Fahrenheit.

In a medium bowl, toss cauliflower with 1/8 teaspoon of salt, cumin and oil. Transfer the mixture to a small baking dish. Place on the oven and roast for 12- 15 minutes or until the cauliflower is tender.

As the cauliflower roasts, you can be making the dressing. Whisk a combination of za'atar, garlic, lemon juice, tahini, water and the remaining salt in a small bowl.

Place the kale in the bottom of a shallow serving bowl and top it with cauliflower, chick peas, quinoa and drizzle the mix with 2 tablespoons of dressing.

Serve and enjoy.

Conclusion

We have come to the end of the book. Thank you for reading and congratulations for reading until the end.

Your struggle to lose weight is not an unsolvable situation. It has a natural solution and that is you rectifying your hormonal imbalance through changing your way of eating. To benefit from this solution, you will need to read and follow every advice you have been given in this book. So I encourage you to start today and you won't regret.

If you found the book valuable, can you recommend it to others? One way to do that is to post a review on Amazon.

Please leave a review for this book on Amazon!

Thank you and good luck!

www.ingramcontent.com/pod-product-compliance
Lightning Source LLC
Chambersburg PA
CBHW022111170526
45157CB00004B/1580